Cooking Down South with Sherry

Lovingly preserved and edited by her son, Todd Thorne

Sherry Thorne

Ada Forge Books

Dedication:

I would like to dedicate this to my niece, Stacy. I promised it to her as a wedding present—though I guess I'm a little late.

I also want to dedicate this to my sister, Linda (Linny), who helped me and encouraged me to see it through.

Sherry Fitzgerald Thorne

Sherry & Cooking
By Todd Thorne

Introduction

By Todd Thorne

Growing up in our house meant dinner was on the table at 6:00 p.m. sharp. Every evening, the family gathered—not just to eat, but to talk about the day, to laugh, to share, and to enjoy the meal that Mom had so lovingly prepared. Sundays were an entire event. Whether it was a potluck at church or a big Sunday meal after the morning service, Mom made sure it was memorable. Saturdays meant breakfast for everyone. And holidays? Holidays were feasts—plates piled high and hearts even fuller—as she cooked for every member of our extended family.

Special moments always had their own special cake. That was how she showed her love. Through food. Through the sound of a spoon against a bowl. Through the smell of something sweet baking in the oven. Cooking wasn't just what she did, it was who she was.

She started young. Her parents both worked, and her mother ran a beauty salon when most women didn't work outside the home. That meant Mom, still just a girl, stepped into the kitchen and began learning by doing. She became the family cook out of necessity, but as the years passed, it became a passion. She didn't just make food; she made memories.

Mom was not a professional chef. She wasn't a food writer. She was a home cook and a baker, the kind who made magic from scratch and never needed a measuring cup to get it right. The recipes in this book may not be perfect, because she wasn't perfect. She was real. She was Momma. She was ours.

For most of her life, she talked about putting together a cookbook. It was always something she planned to do "one day." But it wasn't until the early stages of dementia set in that she made it a priority. She knew the time to preserve those memories was now. So she sat down in her small kitchen and typed each recipe out on her laptop. One by one, with patience and love, she documented the meals that had filled so many bellies and warmed so many hearts.

She compiled the book herself, then took it to a local print shop to have it made into something real, something lasting. She didn't publish it or sell it. She handed it out to us, her family, because we were the ones she made all those meals for. Because we were her purpose. And this was her gift.

As her son, I edited this public edition. I cleaned up the formatting, corrected typos, and standardized punctuation, but these are still Momma's words. Her voice. Her touch. Her story.This cookbook is more than just recipes. It's the story of a woman who loved through butter and sugar, cornbread and gumbo. It's the legacy of a mother who made sure we were always fed, body and soul. And now, it's preserved, just like she hoped.

Sherry's youngest, Todd.

Precious Children

Children Learn What They Live

BY DOROTHY LAW NOLTE, Ph.D.

If children live with **criticism**,
they learn to **condemn**.

If children live with **hostility**,
they learn to **fight**.

If children live with **ridicule**,
they learn to be **shy**.

If children live with **shame**,
they learn to feel **guilt**.

If children live with **tolerance**,
they learn to be **patient**.

If children live with **encouragement**,
they learn **confidence**.

If children live with **praise**,
they learn to **appreciate**.

If children live with **fairness**,
they learn **justice**.

If children live with **security**,
they learn to have **faith**.

If children live with **approval**,
they learn to **like themselves**.

If children live with **acceptance and friendship**,
they learn to find **love** in the world.

Contents

1. Note To Readers 1

* = Check Notes

2. Helpful Hints 5

Tips by Sherry

Drinks

Vegetables

Breads

Desserts

Meats

This and That

3. Section One 11

Main Dishes

1 Fried Chicken

2 Oven Fried Chicken

3 Skillet Pies

4 Chicken and Noodles

5 Chicken Spaghetti

6 Gumbo
7 Baked Chicken or Turkey
8 Aunt Modean's Stuffed Dumplings
9 Chicken Casserole
10 Giblet Gravy
11 Cornbread Dressing
12 Breasts Baked in Mushroom Sauce
13 Hot Chicken Salad Casserole
14 Chicken and Dumplings
15 Squirrel with Brown Dumplings
16 Hobo Beans
17 Teriyaki Chicken
18 Liver and Onions
19 Baked Chicken
20 Shrimp Creole
21 Shrimp Étouffée
22 Hamburger Steaks
23 Dirty Rice
24 Taco Casserole
4. Section Two 53
Salads & Slaws
25 Wilted Salad
26 Coleslaw

27 Overnight Salad
28 Chicken Salad
29 Potato Salad
30 Carrot-Raisin Salad
31 Green Pea Salad
5. Section Three 63
Vegetables & Sides
32 Dry Beans
33 Bean Dumplings
34 Corn Pudding
35 Candied Sweet Potatoes
36 Fried Green Tomatoes
37 Green Peas & Potatoes
38 Broccoli Casserole
39 Green Bean Casserole
40 Sweet Potato Casserole
41 Mixed Squash Casserole
42 Tater Tot Casserole
43 Canned Green Beans
44 Turnip Greens and Corn Dodgers
6. Section Four 82
Bread & Muffins
45 BISCUITS

46 MEXICAN CORNBREAD

47 BANANA BREAD

48 LEMON GLAZED BREAD

49 BLUEBERRY MUFFINS

50 MONKEY BREAD

51 HOT WATER CORNBREAD

52 CAN BISCUIT CINNAMON ROLLS

53 CAN BISCUIT DONUTS

54 MAMA PETTY'S HUSH PUPPIES

55 IRISH SODA BREAD

56 PUMPKIN BREAD

57 SWEET APPLE QUICK BREAD

58 DATE NUT BREAD

7. Section Five 106

Cakes

Classic-Cake Recipes Collection

59 Strawberry Angel Food Cake

60 Easy Cake

61 Grandma Petty's Stack Cake

62 German Chocolate Upside Down Cake

63 Fruit Cake

64 Ultimate Carrot Cake

65 Chewy Cake

66 Italian Cream Cake
67 Lemon-Jello Cake
68 Mandarin-Orange Cake
69 Mississippi-Mud Cake
70 Orange Slice Cake
71 Moist Pineapple Cake
72 Blueberry Pound Cake
73 Fresh Apple Cake
74 Better Than Everything Cake
75 Baked Apple Squares
76 Lemon Pound Cake
77 Honey Bun Cake
78 Baked Cheesecake
79 Orange Cake
80 Tunnel of Fudge Cake

8. Section Six 151

Deserts & Pies

82 Easy Apple Dumplings
83 Bread Pudding with Lemon Sauce
84 Butternut Brownie Pie
85 Pecan Pie
86 Pie Crust for Single Pie
87 Blind bake

88 Best-Ever Apple Pie
89 Hot Apple Toddy
90 Fried Apple Pies
91 Pastry (Double Pie Crust)
92 Banana Pudding (Custard-Based)
93 Cold Banana Pudding
94 Four Layer Delight
95 Shoney's Strawberry Pie
96 Louisiana Tater Pie
97 Coconut Custard Pie (Diabetic-Friendly)
98 Dieter's Pie Crust
99 Apple Pie
100 Tapioca Pudding
101 Strawberry Cheesecake
102 Whoopie Pies
103 Blueberry Pudding Cake
104 Old Time Rice Pudding
105 Cherry Coffee Cake
106 Shortbread Cookies
107 Tea Scones

9. Index 199

Acknowledgements 206

About the author 208

Note To Readers

* = Check Notes

Note to Readers:

Crisco was a staple in Southern kitchens for much of the 20th century, prized by older cooks for its reliability and versatility. Introduced in 1911, this solid vegetable shortening replaced lard in many homes and became the go-to for making the flakiest pie crusts, the crispiest fried chicken, and the most tender biscuits. For many Southern women, a can of Crisco sat proudly on the counter, ready for everything from greasing pans to baking cakes. New cooks today might not reach for it as often, but understanding how it was used can help recreate that unmistakable texture and flavor of vintage recipes. When a recipe calls for Crisco, you can use modern vegetable shortening, or if you prefer, swap in butter or lard, but know that Crisco helped define the soul of Southern cooking for generations.

Oleo, short for oleomargarine, was a household name in Southern kitchens, especially during the Great Depression and wartime years when butter was scarce or expensive. It was an affordable butter substitute made from vegetable oils, and many older recipes passed down through families call for it by name. Cooks of the time used oleo in everything from cakes to cornbread, and it became part of the rhythm of daily life. Today, most people simply call it margarine, and you can easily substitute modern margarine or even butter, depending on your preference. Understanding what oleo was helps preserve the spirit of those cherished recipes, reminding us of the resourcefulness and warmth that filled our grandmothers' kitchens.

Sucaryl was a popular artificial sweetener used in mid-century kitchens, especially by Southern cooks looking to cut down on sugar for health or dietary reasons. Made from cyclamate, it offered a calorie-free option that tasted surprisingly close to sugar. You'll often find it listed in older diabetic-friendly or "diet" recipes from the 1950s and 60s. Though Sucaryl was eventually banned in the United States in 1969 because of health concerns, it remains available in some countries today. For modern cooks, any zero-calorie sweetener, like Stevia, Splenda, or monk fruit can be used in its place. If a vintage recipe calls for Sucaryl, consider it a glimpse into a time when convenience and health-consciousness were just beginning to shape Southern home cooking.

Cheez-Whiz burst onto the scene in the 1950s as a processed cheese spread that quickly found its way into casseroles, dips, and sandwiches across the South. It was prized for its smooth texture, long shelf life, and meltability, making it a go-to shortcut for busy home cooks and potluck favorites. Whether spooned over broccoli, stirred into macaroni, or used as a dip with chips or celery sticks, Cheez Whiz added a creamy, salty kick that defined many comfort-food dishes of the era. While today's cooks might opt for fresh cheeses or homemade sauces, Cheez Whiz still holds a place in vintage recipes and in the memories of those who grew up watching their mothers stir it into bubbling casseroles on a weeknight. If your recipe calls for Cheez Whiz, you can use it as written or substitute with a homemade cheese sauce if you're feeling fancy.

Oak Grove Gumbo Mix is a beloved shortcut for making traditional Cajun-style gumbo, especially popular with Southern home cooks looking for that rich, dark roux flavor without the time or trouble of stirring it from scratch. Sold in a box and made in Louisiana, this mix typically includes a pre-made roux blend of flour and oil, along with seasonings like onion, garlic, and bell pepper. It became a go-to for weeknight meals, church suppers, and family gatherings, just add meat or seafood, water, and let it simmer. While some gumbo purists insist on homemade roux, Oak Grove offers a reliable, flavorful base that delivers that down-home taste with half the effort. If you can't find it locally, you can substitute with a jarred roux or make your own, but for many cooks, Oak Grove brings back the flavor of mama's gumbo pot like nothing else.

Sifting flour was once a standard step in almost every baking recipe, especially in Southern kitchens where biscuits, cakes, and cornbread were everyday fare. The process lightens the flour by breaking up clumps and dispersing ingredients like baking powder or salt when they're mixed in. Older recipes often call for "sifted flour," not just to measure accurately but to help create tender, fluffy textures. While modern pre-packaged flour is finer and more consistent than in decades past, sifting still makes a difference in delicate baked goods. If a recipe says to sift, it's worth the extra minute, especially if you want your biscuits to rise high or your pound cake to feel like a cloud. For today's cook, a fine-mesh strainer works just as well as a sifter, and a quick pass-through can be the secret behind that perfect Southern crumb.

Helpful Hints

Tips by Sherry

Drinks

- Add sparkle to iced fruit juice with calorie-free club soda, it cuts sweetness and calories.

- Always use cold water in electric drip coffee makers. Measure 1–2 tablespoons of ground coffee per cup of water.

Vegetables

- Save water and veggie scraps after cooking, freeze them. Once full, add tomato juice and seasoning for a delicious, homemade soup base.

- Thicken soups and stews easily with a spoonful of instant potatoes.

- Drop a lettuce leaf into hot soup to soak up

grease. Remove before serving. Or refrigerate overnight and skim hardened fat before reheating.

- Cut cabbage and cauliflower odors by adding a splash of vinegar to the water, avoid overcooking.

- Adding three large stalks of chopped celery to about two cups of beans, This helps digestion.

- Rinse hard-boiled eggs in cold water immediately for easy peeling. A drop of food coloring can help you tell. Is it cooked or not?

- Cook pasta for salads until al dente so it absorbs dressing without becoming mushy.

- Prevent oil splatter by sprinkling a little salt or flour into the pan before frying.

- To stop pasta from boiling over, lay a wooden spoon or fork across the top of the pot.

- Store dry pasta, white rice, and grains in airtight containers in a cool, dry place. Refrigerate brown rice, and freeze other grains if not used within five months.

- A few drops of lemon juice added to rice keeps grains separate.
- To prevent beans or corn from becoming tough, add salt halfway through cooking.
- When cooking greens, a teaspoon of sugar helps preserve bright green color.
- Add vinegar or lemon juice to potatoes before draining to make them extra white.

Breads

- Use shortening—not margarine or oil—to grease pans for bread baking.
- When unsure, always sift flour before measuring.
- Lower oven temperature by 25°F when baking in glass pans.
- Store nuts in the freezer. They crack easier when frozen and can be used directly.
- Dust bread pans or counters with flour using a repurposed salt shaker.

- Freeze overripe bananas in a plastic bag until ready to bake banana bread.
- Test egg freshness by placing them in cold water, discard if they float.

Desserts

- Let eggs reach room temperature before whipping, this gives meringues more volume.

Meats

- Parboil meats like ribs or pot roast before grilling to reduce fat.
- Use a plastic bag for easy, mess-free marinating.
- For thin meat slices, partially freeze before cutting.
- Add tomatoes to roasts, natural acid helps tenderize the meat.
- Always thaw meat in the refrigerator for safety.

- Fry chicken in canola oil for a lighter flavor.
- One pound of boneless chicken yields about 3 cups cubed.
- Use a spoon for scalloped edges on pie crusts, or a fork for decorative patterns.
- For a glossy cake finish, gently melt the frosting with a hair dryer.

This and That

- To avoid tearing up when chopping onions, cut them under cold water or chill them briefly in the freezer first.
- Rub lemon juice on hands or counters to remove fish and onion odors.
- Clean Corning Ware by filling it with water and dropping in two denture tablets. Let it sit for 30–45 minutes.
- Add raw rice to salt shakers to prevent clumping.
- Mix 6 parts salt to 1 part pepper in a shaker for

quick table seasoning.

- Need a fast ice pack? A bag of frozen peas does the trick.

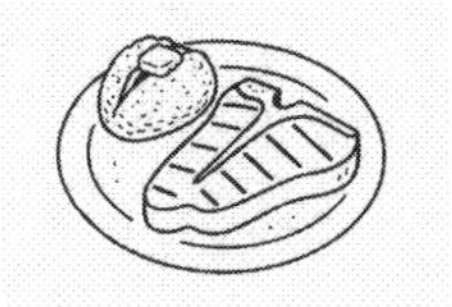

Section One

Main Dishes

1 Fried Chicken

If you like fried chicken, invest in an iron skillet chicken fryer. You will use it for many dishes. When I was growing up, someone in the church would always have the preacher over for Sunday dinner. It was always fried chicken, usually the only fresh meat on hand. There is nothing better than fried chicken made by a good Southern Baptist lady.

Ingredients:

- 1 whole chicken, cut up

- Flour
- Cooking oil
- Salt
- Pepper

Instructions:

1. Fill a deep iron skillet about 1/3 full with oil and heat on medium-high.
2. Wash chicken pieces, then salt and pepper each one.
3. Place flour in a plastic bag, add chicken, and shake well to coat.
4. Place chicken into hot oil. Pack closely.
5. Cook for a few minutes, then cover with a lid. Turn after 10 minutes.
6. Monitor heat level. Chicken should be finished in 20 minutes.

2 Oven Fried Chicken

Ingredients:

- 2 Tbsp butter
- 2 Tbsp oil
- 1 cup flour
- 2 tsp salt
- 2 tsp paprika
- ¼ tsp pepper
- 2 eggs
- ½ cup milk
- Bread crumbs
- 1 cut-up fryer chicken

Instructions:

1. Preheat the oven to 400°F. Add butter and oil to a shallow pan and heat.

2. Mix flour, salt, paprika, and pepper. Coat chicken in mixture.

3. Beat eggs and milk. Dip chicken, then roll in bread crumbs.

4. Place on an oiled baking sheet. Bake for 30 minutes, turn, and continue baking until done.

Other Variations:

- Dip chicken in milk, then in cornflake crumbs. Bake on a cookie sheet.

- Coat chicken with butter or oil, then dip in bread or cornflake crumbs before baking.

3 Skillet Pies

Dough Ingredients:

- 2¾ cups flour
- 2 tsp salt
- ½ cup oil
- ½ cup milk

Instructions:

1. Mix flour and salt. Pour oil into milk (do not stir).
2. Add to flour and stir until mixed. Shape into a ball.
3. Roll dough to ⅛ inch thick. Cut into 5-inch squares.
4. Add a spoonful of filling. Fold to form a triangle. Seal edges with a floured fork.
5. Fry in 1 inch of oil at 350°F for 4–5 minutes, turning to brown both sides. Drain and serve

hot. Can also be baked.

Filling Ingredients:

- ½ cup thick white sauce
- 2 cups chopped chicken
- ¼ cup pimientos
- ¼ tsp pepper *Optional: chopped mushrooms

4 Chicken and Noodles

Ingredients:

- 1 can cream of chicken soup
- ⅓ cup grated Parmesan cheese
- 2 cups cubed cooked chicken
- ½ cup milk
- ⅛ tsp pepper
- 3 cups cooked medium noodles

Instructions:

1. Combine soup, milk, cheese, and pepper in a saucepan.
2. Add noodles and chicken. Heat over low, stirring often.

5 Chicken Spaghetti

Ingredients:

- 2 large onions, chopped
- 2 bell peppers, chopped
- 3 stalks celery, chopped
- 1 bunch green onions, chopped
- ¼ cup chopped parsley
- 4 cloves garlic, chopped
- Deboned chicken
- ¼ cup Worcestershire sauce
- Chicken broth (enough to float ingredients)

Instructions:

1. Saute onions, peppers, celery, and green onions in oil.
2. Add parsley, garlic, chicken, Worcestershire,

and broth. Simmer for 1 hour, adding broth as needed.

3. Boil 12 oz spaghetti in chicken broth. Drain and combine with chicken mixture. Serve immediately. *Note: The chicken mixture can be made ahead and frozen.*

6 Gumbo

Ingredients:

- Cooked chicken
- 2 chopped purple onions
- 2 large cans tomatoes
- 1 package gumbo mix (Oak Grove* or Tony Chachere's)
- 3 cups okra
- Salt and pepper

Instructions:

1. Saute onion and bell pepper. Optional: add hot pepper.
2. Combine cooked chicken broth with tomatoes, onions, peppers, and okra.
3. Cook for 30 minutes. Add chicken or shrimp and gumbo mix.

4. Add tomato sauce and water if needed. Simmer until rice is tender.

7 Baked Chicken or Turkey

Instructions:

1. Salt the bird all over and place in a roasting pan with 1 cup water.

2. Pour 1 stick melted butter over the bird and cover with foil.

3. Bake at 350°F: 1.5 hours for chicken, 3–4 hours for turkey (until the leg moves easily).

4. Uncover for the last 30 minutes to brown.

8 Aunt Modean's Stuffed Dumplings

Ingredients:

- 2 or 3 chicken breasts
- 2 cans cream of chicken soup
- 2 cans cream of mushroom soup
- Water (as needed)
- 4 cans biscuits
- 1 package French onion soup mix

Instructions:

1. Cook chicken in a large pot of water until tender. Remove and let cool. Reserve broth.
2. Mix both soups with enough reserved broth to thin slightly.
3. Shred rested chicken.
4. Flatten biscuits, place chicken on one side, fold

over, and pinch closed.

5. Drop dumplings into boiling soup mix. Continue with all biscuits. Add broth as needed.

9 Chicken Casserole

Ingredients:

- 3 Tbsp butter
- 1½ cups milk or chicken broth
- ¾ cup pre-cooked rice
- 1½ cups bite-sized chicken
- 1 small can of mushrooms with juice
- 1 tsp grated onion
- 1 cup bread crumbs
- 2 Tbsp flour
- 1 cup grated cheese
- 1 package slivered almonds
- 1 cup chopped pimiento

Instructions:

1. Layer ingredients in a casserole dish.

2. Top with bread crumbs and almonds.

3. Bake at 350°F for 20 minutes.

10 Giblet Gravy

Instructions:

1. Boil the neck, giblets, onion, and celery until reduced to a third.

2. Chop giblets and 1 boiled egg.

3. Brown flour in melted shortening or bacon grease.

4. Add broth mixture and stir. Simmer until thickened.

11 Cornbread Dressing

Ingredients:

- 1 cup chopped onion
- ½ stalk celery, chopped
- Pan of cornbread
- 2–3 slices white bread
- 2 cans chicken broth

Instructions:

1. Crumble cornbread and bread slices in a large bowl.
2. Add onion, celery, salt, and pepper.
3. Pour in broth and mix until slightly soupy.
4. Bake at 375°F for about 45 minutes or until brown on top.

12 Breasts Baked in Mushroom Sauce

Ingredients:

- 8 boneless chicken breasts
- Garlic salt
- Paprika
- 1 can cream
- Salt
- 1 can cream of mushroom soup
- 1 can sliced mushrooms (optional)

Instructions:

1. Preheat the oven to 350°F.
2. Sprinkle both sides of chicken with garlic salt, paprika, and salt.
3. Arrange chicken, skin-side up, in a 9x13-inch baking dish.

4. Mix soup and cream, pour over chicken.
5. Bake uncovered for 1 hour or until chicken is tender.
6. Serve with cooked long grain and wild rice.

13 Hot Chicken Salad Casserole

Ingredients:

- 2 cups diced cooked chicken
- 2 ups chopped celery
- ½ cup blanched, chopped salted almonds
- ½ tsp salt
- 1 cup mayonnaise
- 2 Tbsp lemon juice
- ⅓ cup chopped green pepper
- 2 Tbsp chopped pimiento
- 2 cups crushed potato chips
- ⅓ cup grated cheese

Instructions:

1. Blend chicken, celery, almonds, green pepper, pimiento, onion, salt, lemon juice, and mayon-

naise.

2. Layer chicken mixture and crushed chips in a greased 2½-quart casserole.

3. Top with remaining chips and cheese.

4. Bake at 350°F for 20–25 minutes, until the cheese is melted.

14 Chicken and Dumplings

Ingredients:

- 3 to 4 lb chicken
- 2 cups flour
- ¾ cup chicken broth (or as needed)

Instructions:

1. Wash chicken and cover with water in a large pot. Bring to a boil.
2. Reduce heat, cover, and simmer until chicken is tender. Do not overcook.
3. Drain and reserve broth. Cut chicken into chunks.
4. In a bowl, mix flour and enough broth to form a firm but pliable dough.
5. Roll dough and cut into strips.
6. Bring broth to a rolling boil. Add dumplings one at a time.

7. Reduce heat and stir often. Add chicken back in.

15 Squirrel with Brown Dumplings

Ingredients:

- 2 or 3 squirrels (wild game)
- Flour
- Oil (about 1 cup)
- Salt and pepper

For the Roux:

- Reserved oil from frying
- Additional flour
- Water (to create gravy)

Instructions:

1. Flour the squirrels and fry in about 1 cup of oil until browned. Remove and set aside.
2. Drain most of the oil, reserving a few table-

spoons.

3. Add flour to the oil to make a roux. Stir until brown.

4. Add water to the roux to make a gravy. Return squirrels to the pan.

5. Make dumplings separately and add to the gravy.

6. Simmer everything together until the squirrel is tender.

16 Hobo Beans

Ingredients:

- 2 (16 oz) cans Pork n' Beans
- ½ cup water
- 2 Tbsp brown sugar
- 1 cup ketchup
- 1 lb hamburger meat
- 1 chopped onion
- 2 tsp vinegar
- 2 tsp mustard
- 1 can kidney beans

Instructions:

1. Brown hamburger meat and drain.
2. Mix all ingredients together in a 2½-quart baking dish.

3. Cover and bake at 400°F for 30 minutes.

4. This dish can be frozen.

17 Teriyaki Chicken

Ingredients:

- 1 cup ketchup
- ½ cup firmly packed brown sugar
- ½ cup soy sauce
- ¼ cup + 2 Tbsp vegetable oil
- 2 Tbsp cooking sherry
- 6 boneless, skinless chicken breast halves

Instructions:

1. In a bowl, whisk ketchup, brown sugar, soy sauce, ¼ cup oil, and sherry.
2. Pour into a gallon-size zip bag. Add chicken, seal, and refrigerate for at least 2 hours, turning occasionally.
3. Drain chicken and discard marinade.
4. Heat remaining 2 Tbsp oil in a skillet over

medium heat.

5. Cook chicken 5 minutes on each side or until cooked through.

6. Serve with rice.

18 Liver and Onions

Ingredients:

- 2¼ lbs beef liver
- 2 Tbsp margarine
- 2 large eggs
- 3 cups fine dry bread crumbs
- ½ tsp seasoned salt
- 1 cup milk
- 1 large onion, sliced into ¼-inch rings
- 2 Tbsp vegetable oil

Instructions:

1. Soak liver in cold salted water for 15–20 minutes.
2. Melt margarine in a skillet. Cook onion until tender and lightly browned. Sprinkle it with salt and keep warm.

3. Whisk milk and eggs in a bowl. Place bread crumbs in a separate bowl.

4. Rinse and dry liver. Dip in milk mixture, then bread crumbs.

5. Heat oil in a skillet and fry liver 2–3 minutes per side until cooked through.

6. Top with sauteed onions.

19 Baked Chicken

Ingredients:

- 2¼ to 2½ lb chicken
- 1 stick oleo* (melted)
- 1 tsp seasoned salt

Instructions:

1. Preheat the oven to 400°F.
2. Cut chicken in half along backbone and breastbone.
3. Rinse and pat dry. Tuck wings under and place in a baking pan.
4. Brush with butter and sprinkle with seasoned salt.
5. Bake 50–60 minutes, basting with butter throughout.

20 Shrimp Creole

Ingredients:

- 1½ cups chopped onion
- 1 cup chopped celery
- 1 medium green bell pepper, chopped
- 2 minced garlic cloves
- ¼ cup butter or margarine
- 14–16 oz medium shrimp
- 1 (15 oz) can tomato sauce, 1 cup water
- 2 tsp parsley
- 1 tsp salt
- ⅛ tsp cayenne pepper
- 2 crushed bay leaves

Instructions:

1. Saute onion, celery, pepper, and garlic in butter

until tender.

2. Stir in tomato sauce, water, and seasonings. Simmer uncovered for 10 minutes.

3. Add shrimp and simmer covered for 10–20 minutes until shrimp is pink and tender.

4. Serve over 3 cups of cooked rice.

21 Shrimp Étouffée

Ingredients:

- 1½ to 2 lbs peeled shrimp
- 6 Tbsp butter or margarine
- 1 large onion, chopped
- 1 large bell pepper, chopped
- ½ cup chopped celery
- 2–3 Tbsp cornstarch
- 1¾ cups water
- ¼ tsp garlic salt
- 1½ Tbsp tomato paste
- Salt, black pepper, and red pepper to taste

Instructions:

1. Saute onion, pepper, and celery in butter until tender.

2. Stir in seasonings and dissolve cornstarch in part of the water.

3. Add to the skillet and stir until thickened.

4. Add remaining water, tomato paste, and shrimp. Simmer for 20 minutes.

22 Hamburger Steaks

Ingredients:

- 1 lb ground chuck. Salt and pepper
- 1 chopped onion.   2 Tbsp flour

Instructions:

1. Form ground chuck into 5 patties.
2. Fry in a skillet on medium heat until browned on both sides. Remove and set aside.
3. Saute onions in the remaining grease.
4. Add flour to the grease to make a roux. Brown it.
5. Pour in about 2 cups of water and stir to make gravy.
6. Return patties to the pan and simmer for about 45 minutes.

23 Dirty Rice

Ingredients:

- 1 cup rice
- 6 oz chicken livers
- 1½ tsp seasoned salt
- ¾ tsp garlic powder
- 1 cup oleo* (melted)
- ¾ cup chopped onion
- ½ tsp pepper
- ½ cup chopped green onions

Instructions:

1. Cook rice according to package directions.
2. While rice cooks, preheat the oven to 350°F.
3. Place chicken livers in a lightly greased baking pan.

4. Sprinkle 1 tsp salt and ¼ tsp garlic powder. Drizzle with half the melted butter.

5. Bake for 12 minutes, turn, and bake 8–10 more minutes until done.

6. Coarsely chop the livers, reserving any pan liquid.

7. Saute chopped onion in remaining butter until tender.

8. Add the rest of the garlic powder, livers, and reserved liquid. Heat through.

9. Combine with hot cooked rice and mix well.

24 Taco Casserole

Ingredients:

- 1 large bag Doritos chips
- 1 large jar taco sauce
- 1 chopped onion
- 1 lb ground chuck
- 1 can mushroom soup
- Cheddar cheese

Instructions:

1. Brown ground chuck with onion. Drain excess grease.
2. Add taco sauce and mushroom soup. Mix well.
3. In a 9x12-inch casserole dish, layer Doritos, meat mixture, and cheese. Repeat, ending with cheese on top.
4. Cover with foil and bake for 35 minutes at

350°F.

5. Remove foil and bake for 10 more minutes.
6. Serve with shredded lettuce, chopped tomatoes, and sour cream, Serve over rice.

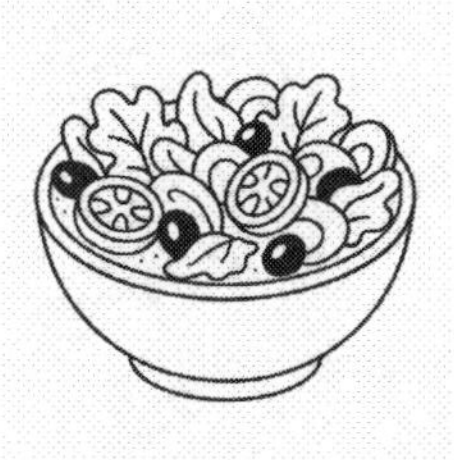

Section Two

Salads & Slaws

25 Wilted Salad

Ingredients:

- 1 large head green leaf lettuce, torn
- 2 boiled eggs, sliced
- 1 bunch green onions, chopped
- Bacon, fried and crumbled

Instructions:

1. Fry bacon in a large skillet until crisp. Remove and crumble.

2. Remove skillet from heat.

3. In the warm skillet (off the burner), layer the lettuce, eggs, and green onions.

4. Top with crumbled bacon and serve immediately.

Memory Note: This was one of our favorites growing up. We raised everything that went into it, and it was always best with pork chops and peas. I'd eat so much I'd get sick, but it was worth it!

26 Coleslaw

Ingredients:

- 1 head cabbage, shredded
- 2 Tbsp sugar
- 1 tsp salt
- Black pepper, to taste
- Mayonnaise (to preference)
- Mustard (a small squirt)

Instructions:

1. Shred cabbage into a large bowl.
2. Sprinkle it with sugar and salt. Let sit for 30 minutes.
3. Add enough mayonnaise to moisten.
4. Add a small squirt of mustard and stir.
5. Season with pepper and additional salt to taste.

Tip: Adjust mayo and mustard to your own taste.

27 Overnight Salad

Ingredients:

- 1 package miniature marshmallows
- 1 can mandarin oranges, drained
- 1 small can (3½ oz) crushed pineapple, drained
- 1 package shredded coconut
- ¼ tsp salt
- 1 pint sour cream

Instructions:

1. Combine all ingredients in a large bowl.
2. Mix well, cover, and refrigerate overnight.

28 Chicken Salad

Ingredients:

- 2 chicken breasts, boiled and shredded
- Grapes (halved, to taste)
- 1 small can pineapple chunks, drained
- Walnuts, chopped
- Salt and pepper, to taste
- Mayonnaise (enough to coat)

Instructions:

1. Boil chicken until cooked through. Cool and shred.
2. Mix with pineapple, grapes, and walnuts.
3. Stir in mayonnaise until well coated.
4. Season to taste.

Serving Suggestion: Great on its own or served on a bed of lettuce for a light dinner.

29 Potato Salad

Ingredients:

- 5 medium potatoes, peeled and diced
- 3 boiled eggs, chopped
- 3 Tbsp sweet pickle relish
- 4 Tbsp mayonnaise
- Squirt of mustard

Instructions:

1. Boil potatoes and eggs until tender. Drain potatoes while still warm.
2. Dice eggs and mix with warm potatoes.
3. Add relish, mayo, and mustard. Stir well.
4. Serve warm or refrigerate until ready.

Tip: Don't let the potatoes cool before mixing—they'll get sticky.

30 Carrot-Raisin Salad

Ingredients:

- 2 lbs carrots, peeled and shredded
- 1 cup raisins
- 1 cup canned crushed pineapple, drained
- 1 cup mayonnaise
- ½ cup powdered sugar

Instructions:

1. In a large bowl, combine carrots, raisins, and pineapple.
2. In a separate bowl, mix mayonnaise and powdered sugar.
3. Pour dressing over carrot mixture and toss to coat.
4. Refrigerate for at least 2 hours.

31 Green Pea Salad

Ingredients:

- 2 cans green peas, drained
- ½ cup mayonnaise
- 1 cup diced cheddar cheese
- ½ cup sweet pickle relish
- ½ cup diced onions

Instructions:

1. Combine all ingredients in a medium bowl.
2. Toss gently until evenly coated.
3. Cover and refrigerate for at least 2 hours before serving.

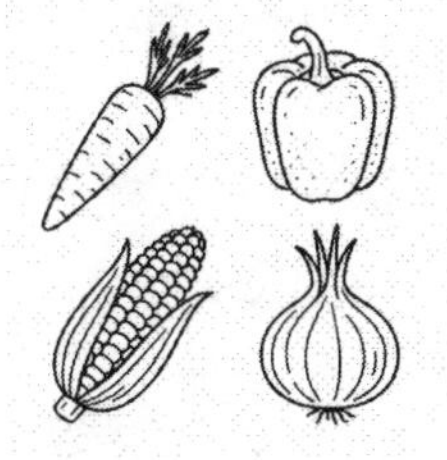

Section Three

Vegetables & Sides

32 Dry Beans

This was a staple in our diet as we were growing up. A sample menu might include:

- Dry salt meat
- Dry Lima beans
- A pan of biscuits
- And sometimes some home fries

Some put syrup in their beans. Others swore by catsup. Sounds good, doesn't it?

Quick Method: The days of all-night soaking and all-day cooking are mostly gone. Here's a shortcut:

- Boil beans in three times as much water as beans for 2 minutes.
- Remove from heat and soak for one hour.
- Always cook beans in the same water they soaked in.
- Add your meat at the start of cooking.
- Add salt when the beans are nearly done.

33 Bean Dumplings

Instructions:

1. Cook beans as directed.
2. Make a simple dough with just flour and milk.
3. Drop spoonfuls into the pot and cook until dumplings are done.

34 Corn Pudding

Ingredients:

- ¼ cup oleo*
- ¼ cup sugar
- 2 cans corn
- ¼ cup flour
- 2 tsp salt
- 3 eggs

Instructions:

1. Melt oleo in a saucepan.

2. Stir in sugar, salt, and flour until smooth.

3. Slowly add milk while stirring.

4. Once thickened, add corn and then eggs.

5. Mix well.

6. Pour into a shallow baking dish

7. Bake at 350°F for 45 minutes or until set.

8. Serve immediately.

35 Candied Sweet Potatoes

A Thanksgiving must-have.

Ingredients:

- 4 lbs sweet potatoes
- 1 cup water
- ½ stick oleo*
- 3½ cups sugar
- ½ cup packed brown sugar

Instructions:

1. Boil potatoes until barely tender.
2. Cool under cold water.
3. Peel and slice ½ inch thick.
4. Layer in a baking dish.
5. Dot with butter and brown sugar.

6. Add water and cover with foil.

7. Bake at 350°F for 1 hour.

36 Fried Green Tomatoes

A Southern tradition.

Ingredients:

- 2 cups flour
- 2½ cups finely crushed saltine crackers
- 1½ cups water
- 1 Tbsp salt
- 6 medium green tomatoes, sliced ¼ inch thick
- Oil for frying

Instructions:

1. Whisk flour, water, and salt in one bowl.
2. Place crumbs in another.
3. Dip tomatoes in flour mixture, then coat with crumbs.

4. Fry in ⅛ inch of hot oil, 2 minutes per side until golden.

37 Green Peas & Potatoes

I remember getting off the school bus at Mama Fitzgerald's house. Terry and I were so hungry. She'd have a pot of peas and potatoes with cornbread and a glass of cold milk. It was *so* good.

Instructions:

1. Shell fresh peas.

2. Wash, and cook in water to cover.

3. Add salt, a bit of butter, and a touch of sugar.

4. For extra goodness, add new potatoes to the pot.

38 Broccoli Casserole

(Thanksgiving favorite)

Ingredients:

- 2 cups cooked rice
- 1 package chopped broccoli
- 1 chopped onion
- 8 oz Cheez Whiz*
- 1 can cream of chicken and mushroom soup
- ½ cup milk
- 3 Tbsp butter
- ¼ cup chopped celery
- ¼ cup chopped onion

Instructions:

1. Sauté celery and onion in butter.

2. Stir in soup, milk, and cheese.

3. Add uncooked, drained broccoli and rice.

4. Mix and pour into a 2-quart casserole.

5. Top with paprika. Bake at 300°F for 30 minutes.

39 Green Bean Casserole

(Another Thanksgiving must)

Ingredients:

- 2 cans green beans, drained
- 1 can French fried onions
- 1 can cream of mushroom soup
- 1 tsp salt
- 1½ cups grated cheddar cheese

Instructions:

1. Mix beans, onions, soup, and salt.
2. Pour into a 2-quart dish.
3. Top with cheese.
4. Bake at 400°F for 30 minutes.

40 Sweet Potato Casserole

Save leftover cornbread—wrap in foil and freeze for dishes like this.

Ingredients:

- 3 cups mashed sweet potatoes
- 2 beaten eggs
- ½ tsp vanilla extract
- 3 Tbsp butter
- ½ cup sugar

Topping:

- ¾ cup brown sugar
- 4 tsp melted butter
- ½ cup flour
- 1 cup chopped pecans

Instructions:

1. Mix sweet potatoes

2. Pour into a buttered casserole dish.

3. Mix topping and sprinkle over top. Bake at 350°F for 20–25 minutes.

41 Mixed Squash Casserole

Leave the skins on! They add color and nutrients.

Ingredients:

- 1 cup sliced carrots
- 4 cups yellow squash, sliced
- 4 cups zucchini, sliced
- ½ cup chopped onion
- 1 tsp salt
- ½ tsp pepper
- ⅔ cup crumbled cornbread
- ⅔ cup torn dry bread
- 1 can cream of chicken soup
- 2 Tbsp oleo*

Instructions:

1. Boil carrots for 6 minutes.

2. Add squash, zucchini, and onion.

3. Simmer for 4 minutes.

4. Drain.

5. Mix soup, salt, pepper, and sour cream.

6. Combine with vegetables and pour into a baking dish.

7. Cover and bake at 350°F for 30 minutes.

8. Top with bread crumbs tossed in butter.

42 Tater Tot Casserole

Ingredients:

- 1 lb ground beef
- 1 small bag tater tots
- 1 can cream of celery soup
- 1 small onion, chopped
- Salt and pepper

Instructions:

1. Preheat the oven to 400°F.
2. Brown beef and onions.
3. Season, then layer in a greased dish.
4. Pour soup over top, then cover with tater tots.
5. Bake for 45 minutes until bubbly.

43 Canned Green Beans

A holiday classic.

Instructions:

1. Fry 6 slices of bacon.

2. Drain 3 large cans of green beans. (save the juice)

3. Fry them in bacon fat.

4. Pour in the reserved juice and simmer.

44 Turnip Greens and Corn Dodgers

Fresh greens are best, but frozen work fine.

Instructions:

1. Wash thoroughly.
2. Boil in a Dutch oven with 1 tsp salt, 1 tsp sugar, and dry salt meat.
3. Cook for 4 hours, adding water as needed for plenty of pot liquor.
4. Mix cornmeal with pot liquor until you have a sticky dough.
5. Rub hands with ice, roll into balls, and drop into the greens.
6. Cook for 20 minutes or until done.

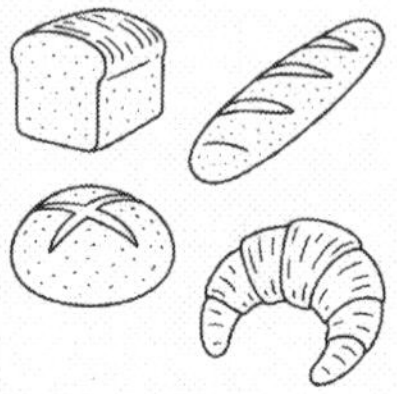

Section Four

Bread & Muffins

45 BISCUITS

When my brother, Terry and I were young, we'd get home from school and grab a cold biscuit. We'd poke a hole in the center, fill it with sugar or syrup, and that was our snack. In the mornings, we'd slice leftover biscuits in half, spread butter, sprinkle sugar, and put them under the broiler to make "biscuit toast." Try it, it's really good.

You can also pour syrup on a plate, add a pat of butter, stir it around, and sop with your biscuit. They're great with gravy, too.

Ingredients:

- Flour (fill a large bowl)
- 1½ cups milk (sweet or buttermilk)
- ½ cup Crisco*
- 2 Tbsp shortening (for skillet)
- Extra flour (for dusting)
- Melted shortening (for topping)

**Note:* *If a recipe calls for Crisco, any solid vegetable shortening will work, but butter or lard can be used instead, depending on the flavor and texture you want*

Instructions:

1. Make a nest in the flour with your hand. Pour in milk and Crisco. Mix with your hand using

a circular motion until the dough is medium firm.

2. Sprinkle the dough with a little flour. Pinch off pieces about the size of an egg and shape by turning under in a circular motion.

3. Place in a heavy pan or iron skillet with 2 tablespoons of shortening.

4. Spoon melted shortening over the top.

5. Bake at 450°F for 18–20 minutes, depending on your oven.

46 MEXICAN CORNBREAD

Ingredients:

- 1 cup cornmeal mix
- 1 cup milk
- 2 eggs
- ½ lb grated cheese
- 1 can cream-style corn
- 1 lb hamburger
- 1 chopped onion
- 1 jalapeño pepper

Instructions:

1. Mix cornmeal, milk, eggs, and corn.
2. Brown meat with onion and pepper.
3. In a greased iron skillet, pour in half the cornmeal mixture.

4. Layer with meat mixture, then cheese, then remaining cornmeal mix.
5. Bake at 350°F for about 30 minutes, or until golden brown.

47 BANANA BREAD

You can freeze overripe bananas and use them later.

Ingredients:

- 2 cups self-rising flour
- 2 eggs
- 1½ cups mashed ripe bananas
- ½ cup butter
- ¾ cup sugar
- ½ cup chopped nuts

Instructions:

1. Beat butter and sugar. Add eggs and bananas. Mix well.
2. Stir in flour. Pour into a greased loaf pan.
3. Bake at 350°F for 1 hour.

48 LEMON GLAZED BREAD

Ingredients:

- ½ cup oil
- 1 cup sugar
- 2 eggs
- 1¼ cups flour
- Grated peel of 1 lemon
- ½ cup milk

Topping:

- ¼ cup sugar
- Juice of 1 lemon

Instructions:

1. Mix bread ingredients. Pour into a greased and floured 9x13-inch pan.
2. Bake at 350°F for 1 hour.

3. While hot, poke holes in the top and pour lemon-sugar topping over.

4. Let cool for 30 minutes before removing from the pan.

49 BLUEBERRY MUFFINS

Ingredients:

- 2 heaping cups self-rising flour
- 1 cup sugar
- 1 cup blueberries
- ½ cup Crisco*
- 1 cup milk
- 1 tsp vanilla

Instructions:

1. Preheat the oven to 425°F.
2. Mix all ingredients except blueberries.
3. Gently fold in blueberries.
4. Fill muffin tins ¾ full. Sprinkle sugar on top.
5. Bake for 20 minutes.

50 MONKEY BREAD

Ingredients:

- 4 cans biscuits
- ½ cup chopped pecans
- ½ cup brown sugar
- 4 Tbsp melted margarine

Separate:

- 1 stick margarine
- 2 tsp cinnamon
- 1 cup sugar

Instructions:

1. Preheat the oven to 350°F.
2. Mix pecans, brown sugar, and melted margarine. Pour into a bundt pan.
3. Mix sugar and cinnamon. Melt margarine.

4. Dip each biscuit in cinnamon sugar, then butter. Layer in pan.
5. Bake for 40 minutes. Cool 20 minutes before serving.

51 HOT WATER CORN-BREAD

A summertime favorite during the hot, humid, days of Summer, made to keep the kitchen cool.

Ingredients:

- 1 cup cornmeal mix
- Boiling water

Instructions:

1. Pour boiling water into cornmeal, stir until sticky.
2. Rub hands with ice to prevent sticking. Pinch off a ball and flatten.
3. Drop into hot oil and fry until golden. (Oil should sizzle when water hits it.)

52 CAN BISCUIT CINNAMON ROLLS

Ingredients:

- 1 can biscuits
- 2 Tbsp cinnamon
- ½ cup sugar
- Cream cheese frosting

Instructions:

1. Place biscuits in a greased round pan.
2. Sprinkle it with sugar and cinnamon mixture.
3. Bake according to package directions.
4. Frost while warm.

53 CAN BISCUIT DONUTS

I always had to make two cans—I'd eat half before the boys got home!

Ingredients:

- 1 can biscuits
- 2 Tbsp milk
- ½ cup powdered sugar

Instructions:

1. Heat oil in a skillet.
2. Punch hole in center of each biscuit.
3. Fry until golden. Mix milk and powdered sugar for glaze.
4. Dip donuts while hot.

54 MAMA PETTY'S HUSH PUPPIES

Ingredients:

- 2 cups cornmeal mix
- 1 cup milk
- 1 finely chopped onion

Instructions:

1. Mix all ingredients.
2. Shape into balls.
3. Fry in medium-hot oil until brown. (Don't let oil get too hot.)

55 IRISH SODA BREAD

Ingredients:

- 4 cups flour
- ¼ cup sugar
- 1 tsp salt
- 1 tsp baking soda
- 1 tsp baking powder
- ¼ cup margarine
- 3 Tbsp caraway seed
- 2 cups raisins
- 1⅓ cups buttermilk
- 2 egg whites, beaten. Milk (for brushing)

Instructions:

1. Combine dry ingredients. Cut in margarine until crumbly.

2. Stir in caraway seeds and raisins.

3. Add buttermilk and egg whites. Stir just until moistened.

4. Knead lightly and shape into a ball. Place on a 7-inch greased pan.

5. Cut a shallow cross on top. Brush with milk. 6. Bake at 375°F for 1 hour.

56 PUMPKIN BREAD

Ingredients:

- 3 cups sugar
- 1 cup oil
- 3 eggs
- ⅔ cup water
- 3 cups flour
- 1 tsp cinnamon
- 1½ tsp salt
- 1 tsp nutmeg
- ½ tsp baking soda
- 1 Tbsp baking powder
- 2 cups pumpkin. 1 cup chopped nuts

Instructions:

1. Beat sugar, oil, and eggs.

2. Sift together dry ingredients. Add alternately with water.

3. Stir in pumpkin and nuts. 4. Pour into greased loaf pans.

4. Bake at 350°F for 90 minutes or until a toothpick comes out clean.

57 SWEET APPLE QUICK BREAD

Ingredients:

- 2 cups flour
- 1 cup sugar
- 1 tsp baking soda
- ½ tsp baking powder
- 1 cup finely chopped apples
- 2 Tbsp corn syrup
- 2 eggs
- ½ cup butter, softened
- ½ cup milk
- 2 Tbsp orange peel. ½ cup chopped nuts

Instructions:

1. Beat all ingredients except nuts for 3 minutes.

2. Fold in nuts. Pour into a greased loaf pan.
3. Bake at 325°F for 50–60 minutes. Cool before slicing.

58 DATE NUT BREAD

Ingredients:

- 2 cups boiling water
- 2½ cups chopped dates
- 2 tsp baking soda
- Dash of salt
- ½ cup sugar
- 2 eggs
- 2 tsp vanilla
- 3 cups flour
- 2 Tbsp melted butter
- 1 cup chopped nuts

Instructions:

1. Pour boiling water over dates. Let sit.
2. Mix soda, sugar, eggs, vanilla, salt, and butter.

3. Add flour, dates with water, and nuts.
4. Pour into two greased loaf pans.
5. Bake at 350°F for 1 hour. Serve with butter or cream cheese.

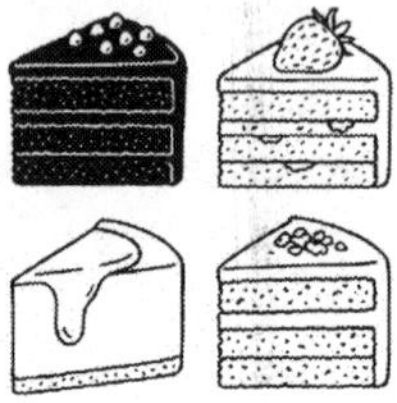

Section Five

Cakes

Classic-Cake Recipes Collection

59 Strawberry Angel Food Cake

This is a great cake to serve in the summer.

Ingredients:

- 1 large angel food cake
- 1 large box strawberry Jello

- 3 cups chopped fresh strawberries or 2 boxes frozen strawberries, drained
- 1 large Cool Whip

Instructions:

1. Cut the top off the cake and set aside.
2. Tear bite-sized pieces from the middle and place in a bowl.
3. Prepare Jello per package directions.
4. Add strawberries; chill to thicken slightly.
5. Fold in cake pieces.
6. Fill hollowed-out cake with mixture.
7. Replace the top.
8. Serve with Cool Whip.
9. Keep refrigerated.

60 Easy Cake

Ingredients:

- 1 Butter Recipe cake mix
- 3/4 cup oil
- 4 eggs
- 1 cup milk
- 1 can coconut pecan frosting (with extra pecans if desired)

Instructions:

1. Mix the first four ingredients on low speed.
2. Beat on medium for 2 minutes.
3. Stir in frosting and pecans.
4. Pour into a greased bundt pan and bake at 325°F for 1 hour.

61 Grandma Petty's Stack Cake

Cake Ingredients:

- 1 package yellow cake mix
- 1 package (3 oz) vanilla pudding mix
- 1 1/3 cups water
- 4 eggs
- 1/4 cup oil
- 2 cups coconut
- 1 cup chopped nuts

Cake Instructions:

1. Blend the first five ingredients.
2. Beat 4 minutes on medium speed.
3. Stir in coconut and nuts.
4. Pour into three greased and floured 9-inch pans.

5. Bake at 350°F for 35 minutes.

6. Cool for 10 minutes, then remove and cool completely.

Frosting Ingredients:

- 4 Tbsp oleo*
- 2 cups coconut
- 8 oz cream cheese
- 3 1/2 cups powdered sugar
- 1/2 tsp vanilla
- 1–2 Tbsp milk

Frosting Instructions:

1. Toast 1 3/4 cups coconut in 2 Tbsp oleo until golden.

2. Cool on a paper towel.

3. Cream remaining oleo and cream cheese.

4. Add milk, then sugar and vanilla.

5. Stir in toasted coconut.

6. Spread between and on cake layers.

7. Sprinkle remaining 1/4 cup coconut on top.

62 German Chocolate Upside Down Cake

Ingredients:

- 1 Can of coconut
- 1 Cup chopped pecans
- German chocolate cake mix
- 1 stick butter
- 8 oz cream cheese
- 1 box powdered sugar

Instructions:

1. Butter and flour a 9x13-inch baking pan.
2. Mix 1 can of coconut with 1 cup chopped pecans; spread in pan.
3. Prepare German chocolate cake mix per box; pour over coconut-pecan layer.
4. Mix 1 stick softened butter, 8 oz cream cheese,

and 1 box powdered sugar.

5. Drop spoonfuls over batter.

6. Bake at 325°F for 1 hour. Cool and invert.

63 Fruit Cake

Made every Christmas, first by Mama, then by me.

Ingredients:

- 1 box vanilla wafers, crushed
- 4 cups chopped pecans
- 1 box raisins
- 1 can sweetened condensed milk

Instructions:

1. Combine all ingredients by hand in a large bowl.
2. Line a tube pan with wax paper.
3. Pack mixture into pan tightly.
4. Cover with wax paper and refrigerate

overnight.

5. Remove from pan and seal.

64 Ultimate Carrot Cake

Ingredients:

- 1 package carrot cake mix
- 1/2 cup water
- 1/2 cup oil
- 4 eggs
- 1 (8 oz) can crushed pineapple with juice
- 1/2 cup chopped nuts
- 1/2 cup coconut
- 1/2 cup raisins
- 1 can cream cheese frosting

Instructions:

1. Preheat the oven to 350°F.

2. Grease and lightly flour two 9-inch pans.

3. Beat mix, water, oil, eggs, and pineapple for 30

sec (low), then 2 min (medium).

4. Stir in nuts, coconut, and raisins.

5. Bake for 40–45 minutes or until the toothpick comes out clean.

6. Cool for 10 minutes in pans, then transfer to racks.

7. Frost cooled cake and refrigerate.

65 Chewy Cake

Ingredients:

- 1 yellow cake mix
- 1 egg
- 1 stick oleo*
- 8 oz cream cheese
- 2 eggs
- 2 cups powdered sugar

Instructions:

1. Preheat oven to 350°F.
2. Grease and flour a baking pan.
3. Mix cake mix, 1 egg, and margarine.
4. Press into the bottom of prepared pan.
5. Mix cream cheese, 2 eggs, and sugar until smooth.

6. Pour over cake base.

7. Bake for 45 minutes.

66 Italian Cream Cake

Colleen Bell made this on my 30th birthday, it was my first birthday cake. Lonny's favorite.

Ingredients:

- 1 stick oleo*
- 1 cup shortening
- 2 cups sugar
- 2 cups flour
- 1 cup buttermilk
- 1 tsp baking soda
- 5 eggs (separated). 1 small can coconut.
- 2 cups ground pecans. 1 tsp vanilla extract

Instructions:

1. Cream shortening and oleo.

2. Add egg yolks one at a time, beating well.
3. Alternate adding flour/soda mix and buttermilk.
4. Beat egg whites until stiff; fold into batter.
5. Fold in coconut and pecans.
6. Pour into 3 greased cake pans.
7. Bake at 350°F for 25–30 minutes.
8. Cool, then frost.

Cream Cheese Frosting:

- 8 oz cream cheese
- 1 stick oleo*
- 1 cup pecans
- 1 box powdered sugar
- 1 tsp vanilla

Cream together until smooth. Frost cake.

67 Lemon-Jello Cake

This is my favorite cake in the world.

Ingredients:

- 1 package lemon cake mix
- 1 package lemon Jello
- 4 eggs
- 3/4 cup water
- 1 cup cooking oil
- 1/2 cup lemon juice
- 2 cups powdered sugar

Instructions:

1. Preheat the oven to 375°F.

2. Mix cake mix, Jello, water, and oil.

3. Pour into a greased bundt pan.

4. Bake for 60 minutes.
5. Pierce hot cake with a fork.
6. Mix lemon juice with powdered sugar and pour over warm cake.

68 Mandarin-Orange Cake

Cake Ingredients:

- 1 package yellow cake mix
- 1/2 cup oil
- 4 eggs
- 1 can (11 oz) mandarin orange slices

Instructions:

1. Beat all ingredients on low speed to combine, then on medium for 2 minutes.
2. Pour into greased pans.
3. Bake at 350°F for 30 minutes or until done.
4. Cool for 10 minutes in pans, then transfer to racks.

Frosting:

- 1 can (20 oz) crushed pineapple, drained

- 1 (9 oz) carton Cool Whip
- 1 box vanilla instant pudding

Instructions:

1. Mix all ingredients together until blended.
2. Chill before spreading on cake.

69 Mississippi-Mud Cake

Cake Ingredients:

- 1 3/4 cups sugar
- 1/3 cup cocoa
- 4 eggs
- 1 1/2 cups flour
- 1 cup oil
- 1 tsp vanilla
- 1 cup nuts
- 1 small package marshmallows

Instructions:

1. Preheat the oven to 350°F.
2. Stir sugar and cocoa together.
3. Add oil, vanilla, and eggs one at a time, mixing well.

4. Add flour and nuts; stir until smooth.

5. Pour into a greased 9x13 pan.

6. Bake until done; top with marshmallows.

7. Return to the oven at 300°F until melted.

8. Let cool.

Icing:

- 1 1/2 sticks oleo*
- 1/2 cup cocoa
- 1 tsp vanilla extract
- 1 box powdered sugar
- 1/4 cup evaporated milk

Mix and spread over cooled cake.

70 Orange Slice Cake

Ingredients:

- 2 sticks oleo*
- 2 cups sugar
- 4 eggs
- 2 cups orange slice candy, chopped
- 1 can coconut
- 1/2 cup buttermilk
- 1 tsp baking soda
- 3 1/2 cups flour
- 1 package dates
- 2 cups chopped nuts
- Dash of salt
- 1 small can crushed pineapple

Instructions:

1. Preheat the oven to 325°F or 350°F.
2. Cream oleo, sugar, and eggs.
3. In a separate bowl, combine flour, soda, and salt.
4. Add dry ingredients to the creamed mixture alternately with buttermilk.
5. Process orange candy with some buttermilk in a food processor.
6. Stir in candy mix, coconut, pineapple, dates, and nuts.
7. Pour into a greased and floured pan.
8. Bake 1 1/2 to 2 hours, or until a toothpick comes out clean.
9. While warm, top with orange juice and powdered sugar.

71 Moist Pineapple Cake

Ingredients:

- 2 cups self-rising flour
- 1 1/2 cups sugar
- 1/2 cup oil
- #2 can crushed pineapple (about 20 oz)
- 2 eggs
- 1 tsp vanilla extract

Instructions:

1. Preheat the oven to 325°F.
2. Mix all ingredients in a large bowl.
3. Pour into a greased oblong baking pan.
4. Bake for 45 minutes.

Icing:

- 1 cup sugar
- 1/2 cup evaporated milk
- 1 stick oleo*
- 1/2 cup chopped nuts
- 1 cup coconut

Instructions:

1. Melt oleo in a saucepan.
2. Add sugar and milk. Cook for 2 minutes.
3. Stir in nuts and coconut.
4. Pour over hot cake.

72 Blueberry Pound Cake

Ingredients:

- 1 yellow cake mix
- 8 oz cream cheese, softened
- 3 eggs
- 15 oz can whole blueberries, drained

Instructions:

1. Preheat the oven to 350°F.
2. Mix cake mix, cream cheese, and eggs until smooth.
3. Gently fold in drained blueberries.
4. Grease and flour a bundt pan.
5. Pour batter into the pan.
6. Bake for 1 hour.
7. Cool for 20 minutes before removing.

73 Fresh Apple Cake

This was Mother's favorite cake.

Ingredients:

- 3 cups chopped tart apples
- 1 cup chopped pecans
- 3 cups flour
- 1 1/2 tsp cinnamon
- 1/4 tsp salt. 1 1/4 cups oil
- 1 1/2 tsp vanilla extract, 2 eggs

Instructions:

1. Preheat the oven to 350°F.
2. Mix flour, cinnamon, salt, oil, and vanilla in a large bowl.
3. In a separate bowl, beat eggs and gradually add sugar until well blended.

4. Fold egg mixture into flour mixture.
5. Stir in apples and pecans (batter will be stiff).
6. Pour into a greased bundt pan.
7. Bake for 1 to 1 1/2 hours, or until the toothpick comes out clean.

74 Better Than Everything Cake

Ingredients:

- 1 yellow cake mix
- 1 cup crushed pineapple
- 1 package instant vanilla pudding mix
- 1 container Cool Whip
- 1 cup sugar
- 2 cups milk
- 2 cups pecans
- 8 oz cream cheese
- 3 ripe bananas. Coconut (to taste)

Instructions:

1. Bake cake as directed in a greased 9x13 pan.
2. Boil sugar and pineapple in a saucepan for 5 minutes.

3. Pour hot mixture over warm cake. Let cool completely.

4. Mix milk, pudding, and softened cream cheese until smooth.

5. Spread pudding mixture over cake.

6. Add sliced bananas. 7. Top with Cool Whip.

8. Sprinkle with coconut and pecans.

75 Baked Apple Squares

Ingredients:

- 1 3/4 cups sugar
- 3 eggs
- 1 tsp cinnamon
- 2 cups thinly sliced apples
- 1 tsp vanilla extract
- 1 cup oil
- 1 cup chopped nuts

Instructions:

1. Preheat the oven to 350°F.
2. Mix all ingredients until well blended.
3. Pour into a greased 9x13 pan.
4. Bake for 40–45 minutes.

76 Lemon Pound Cake

Cake Ingredients:

- 2 cups flour
- 2 cups sugar
- 1 tsp grated lemon peel
- 3 eggs
- 1 tsp vanilla extract
- 2 sticks oleo*
- 1 (8 oz) container pineapple or orange yogurt

Instructions:

1. Preheat the oven to 350°F.
2. Mix all ingredients until well blended.
3. Pour into a greased and floured bundt pan.
4. Bake for 60–70 minutes or until the toothpick comes out clean.

Glaze:

- 1 cup confectioners' sugar
- 1 Tbsp oleo*
- 1–2 Tbsp lemon juice

Mix and pour over the warm cake.

77 Honey Bun Cake

Cake Ingredients:

- 1 yellow cake mix
- 4 eggs
- 8 oz sour cream
- 1/3 cup chopped pecans
- 2 tsp cinnamon
- 2 sticks oleo*, softened
- 1/2 cup brown sugar

Instructions:

1. Preheat the oven to 350°F. Grease a 9x13 pan.
2. Reserve 1/2 cup dry cake mix.
3. Beat remaining mix with oleo, eggs, and sour cream for 2 minutes.
4. Spread half into pan.

5. Mix reserved mix with brown sugar, pecans, and cinnamon.
6. Sprinkle over batter. Drop remaining batter by spoonfuls and spread.
7. Bake for 30–33 minutes.

Glaze:

- Powdered sugar
- Milk
- Vanilla extract

Instructions:

1. Mix until drizzling consistency.
2. Poke warm cake with fork
3. Drizzle glaze over top.
4. Cool completely.

78 Baked Cheesecake

Crust:

- 1 1/2 cups graham cracker crumbs
- 1/4 cup sugar
- 1/4 cup oleo*, melted

Filling:

- 1 1/4 lbs (2 1/2 blocks) cream cheese, softened
- 1 cup sugar
- 3 jumbo eggs
- 1 cup sour cream
- 2 Tbsp plain flour
- 1/2 tsp vanilla extract
- 1/2 tsp lemon juice

Instructions:

1. Mix crust ingredients and press into bottom and 1 inch up sides of 9 inch spring-form pan.

2. Bake the crust at 350°F for 10 minutes; cool completely.

3. Beat cream cheese and sugar until creamy.

4. Add eggs one at a time, mixing well.

5. Add sour cream, flour, vanilla, and lemon juice. Blend gently.

6. Pour into the cooled crust. Bake at 350°F for 30–35 minutes.

7. Cool on a wire rack. Refrigerate for at least 2 hours. Garnish with fruit if desired.

79 Orange Cake

Ingredients:

- 1 box yellow cake mix
- 1 box orange Jello
- 1 1/2 cups butter
- 1/2 tsp orange extract
- Powdered sugar (for garnish)

Instructions:

1. Prepare cake mix per package instructions.
2. Reserve 1 1/2 cups of batter.
3. Mix reserved batter with Jello, butter, and orange extract.
4. Pour plain batter into a greased pan.
5. Spoon orange mixture on top and swirl with fork.

6. Bake at 350°F for 45 minutes.

7. Cool and sprinkle with powdered sugar.

80 Tunnel of Fudge Cake

Cake Ingredients:

- 1 3/4 cups sugar
- 2 cups powdered sugar
- 2 1/4 cups plain flour
- 2 cups chopped walnuts or pecans
- 1 3/4 cups margarine
- 6 eggs
- 3/4 cup unsweetened cocoa

Instructions:

1. Preheat the oven to 350°F. Grease and flour a 12-cup bundt pan.
2. Cream sugar and margarine until fluffy.
3. Add eggs one at a time, beating after each.
4. Gradually add powdered sugar.

5. Stir in flour, cocoa, and nuts by hand.

6. Pour into the pan. Bake for 45–50 minutes.

7. Cool in pan before removing.

Glaze:

- 3/4 cup powdered sugar
- 1/4 cup unsweetened cocoa
- 4–6 tsp milk

Mix to drizzling consistency and pour over cooled cake.

Note: Nuts are essential for the tunnel effect. Walnuts or pecans work best.

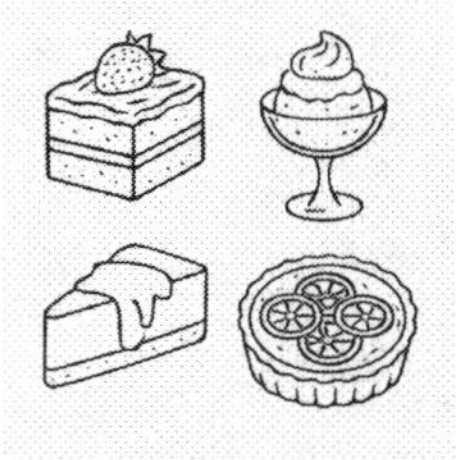

Section Six

Deserts & Pies

81 Lazy Man's Peach Cobbler

Ingredients:

- 1 cup self-rising flour
- 3/4 cup sugar
- 1 cup milk
- 1 stick butter (or oleo*), melted
- 1 large can (29 oz) sliced peaches in juice
- 1 teaspoon vanilla extract

Instructions:

1. Preheat the oven to 375°F.

2. In a medium bowl, whisk together flour, sugar, milk, and vanilla until smooth.

3. Place butter in a 9x13-inch baking dish and melt it in the oven or microwave.

4. Pour the batter over the melted butter—do not stir.

5. Add the peaches with juice into the center of the batter. Do not stir.

6. Bake for 1 hour, or until golden brown and bubbly.

7. Serve hot with a scoop of vanilla ice cream.

82 Easy Apple Dumplings

Ingredients:

- 1 stick butter
- 1 cup sugar
- 1 cup water
- 1 can crescent rolls
- 1 large apple, peeled and sliced into 8 pieces
- Ground cinnamon, for sprinkling

Instructions:

1. Preheat the oven to 375°F.
2. In a saucepan, combine butter, sugar, and water. Bring to a boil and remove from heat.
3. Wrap each apple slice in a crescent roll triangle.
4. Place the wrapped apples in a baking dish.
5. Pour the hot butter-sugar mixture evenly over

the rolls.

6. Sprinkle with cinnamon.
7. Bake for 15 to 18 minutes, or until golden brown.
8. Serve hot with vanilla ice cream.

83 Bread Pudding with Lemon Sauce

Cinnamon Sugar Ingredients:

- 6 tablespoons sugar
- 2 tablespoons cinnamon

Pudding Ingredients:

- 7 jumbo eggs
- 3/4 cup sugar
- 1/2 teaspoon vanilla extract
- 6 to 8 slices day-old white bread, torn into pieces
- 1/4 cup raisins
- 3 cups milk

Lemon Sauce Ingredients:

- 3/4 cup sugar

- 1/2 cup lemon juice
- 2 tablespoons cornstarch
- 1 tablespoon + 1 1/2 teaspoons water

Instructions:

1. Preheat the oven to 350°F.
2. Mix cinnamon and sugar in a small bowl and set aside.
3. In a large bowl, whisk together milk, eggs, sugar, and vanilla.
4. Place torn bread in a 2-quart baking dish. Sprinkle raisins over the bread.
5. Pour the milk mixture over the bread and raisins. Sprinkle it with cinnamon sugar. Cover with foil.
6. Bake for 45 minutes. Remove foil and bake for another 10 minutes until golden.

To make the Lemon Sauce

Instructions:

1. In a small saucepan, combine sugar and lemon juice. Bring to a boil over medium heat.

2. In a separate bowl, dissolve cornstarch in water.

3. Stir the cornstarch mixture into the saucepan. Cook, stirring constantly, until thickened.

4. warm over the bread pudding.

84 Butternut Brownie Pie

Ingredients:

- 4 jumbo egg whites, room temperature
- 1/8 teaspoon baking powder
- 1/8 teaspoon cream of tartar
- 1 1/4 cups sugar
- 14 graham cracker squares, broken into small pieces
- 1 cup pecan pieces
- 1/2 teaspoon vanilla extract
- Cool Whip, for topping
- Chopped pecans, for garnish

Instructions:

1. Preheat the oven to 300°F. Lightly grease a 9-inch pie plate.

2. In a large mixing bowl, beat egg whites and baking powder until soft peaks form.

3. Add cream of tartar and continue beating.

4. Gradually add sugar, one tablespoon at a time, until stiff peaks form.

5. Gently fold in graham cracker and pecan pieces.

6. Spoon into the prepared pie plate and smooth the top.

7. Bake for 30 minutes, or until a wooden pick comes out clean.

8. Cool completely on a wire rack.

9. Top with Cool Whip and sprinkle with chopped pecans. Refrigerate before serving.

85 Pecan Pie

Ingredients:

- 1 cup sugar
- 1 cup light Karo syrup
- 2 tablespoons melted butter (or oleo*)
- 3 jumbo eggs
- 1 cup chopped pecans
- 1 teaspoon vanilla extract
- 1 unbaked pie crust

Instructions:

1. Preheat the oven to 350°F.
2. In a large bowl, combine sugar, Karo syrup, melted butter, eggs, pecans, and vanilla. Mix w ell.
3. Pour into an unbaked pie crust.

4. Bake for 1 hour, or until the filling is set.
5. Let cool before serving. Perfect for Thanksgiving or any holiday table.

86 Pie Crust for Single Pie

Ingredients:

- 1 1/3 cups flour
- 1/2 cup shortening
- 1/2 teaspoon salt
- 3 teaspoons cold milk

Instructions:

1. Sift flour and salt together in a bowl.
2. In a glass measuring cup, mix shortening and cold milk. Beat well.
3. Pour the mixture into the flour and form into a ball.
4. Roll dough between two pieces of wax paper with a rolling pin.
5. Transfer the rolled crust to a pie plate, starting at one side and working across.

87 Blind bake

Instructions:

1. Place wax paper over the crust.
2. Fill with dry beans to weigh it down.
3. Bake at 375°F for about 10 minutes, or until lightly browned.

88 Best-Ever Apple Pie

Ingredients:

- 9-inch double pie crust
- 6 cups tart apples, peeled and sliced
- Dash of nutmeg
- 1/2 cup sugar
- 1/4 cup brown sugar
- 1 tablespoon flour
- 1/2 teaspoon cinnamon

- 1/4 cup butter
- 1 tablespoon milk

Instructions:

1. Preheat the oven to 425°F.
2. Line the bottom of the pie dish with one crust.
3. Arrange sliced apples neatly in the bottom crust.
4. In a bowl, mix sugars, flour, and cinnamon.
5. Sprinkle the mixture evenly over the apples.
6. Dot with butter and dust lightly with nutmeg.
7. Cover with top crust. Brush with milk and sprinkle with sugar.
8. Cut five slits in the top crust to allow steam to escape.
9. Bake for 15 minutes at 425°F, then reduce heat to 350°F and bake for 45 minutes more, or until golden brown.

89 Hot Apple Toddy

Ingredients:

- 1 quart apple cider
- 1/3 cup brown sugar
- 1/2 lemon, sliced
- 1 1/2 tablespoons Southern Comfort

Instructions:

1. In a saucepan, simmer apple cider, brown sugar, and lemon slices for 10 minutes.
2. Stir in Southern Comfort.
3. Serve warm. Excellent for soothing colds and comforting the soul.

90 Fried Apple Pies

Filling Ingredients:

- Dried apple slices
- Water (just enough to cook)
- 1 cup sugar

Instructions:

1. Wash and core the dried apples.
2. Place in a pot with a small amount of water and add sugar.
3. Cook over medium heat until the apples are soft enough to mash with a fork.
4. Continue cooking until the water cooks out.
5. Cool the filling in the refrigerator before using it in pastry.

91 Pastry (Double Pie Crust)

Ingredients:

- 2/3 cup shortening
- 3 to 4 tablespoons water
- 2 cups flour
- 1/4 teaspoon baking powder

Instructions:

1. Mix all ingredients together lightly.
2. Knead dough three times, form into a ball, and let rest for 15–20 minutes.
3. Roll out half the dough at a time to 1/8 inch thickness.
4. Cut into saucer-sized circles.
5. Add filling to one side of each circle, fold over, and pinch edges to seal.
6. In a deep iron skillet, heat about 2 inches of oil.
7. Fry pies until golden brown on both sides.

These pies are rustic, lightly sweet, and full of tradition—perfect warm from the skillet or enjoyed later.

92 Banana Pudding (Custard-Based)

Custard Ingredients:

- 3 eggs, separated
- 3/4 cup sugar
- 4 tablespoons cornstarch
- 2 cups milk
- 1 teaspoon vanilla extract
- 2 tablespoons butter

To Assemble:

- Vanilla wafers
- 3 bananas, sliced

Instructions:

1. In a saucepan, mix milk, cornstarch, egg yolks, and sugar.

2. Cook over medium heat, stirring constantly until thick and bubbly.

3. Remove from heat and stir in vanilla and butter.

4. In a 2-quart dish, layer wafers, bananas, and custard.

5. Repeat layers, ending with custard on top.

Meringue Ingredients:

- 3 egg whites, room temperature
- 6 tablespoons sugar
- 1 teaspoon vanilla extract

Instructions:

1. In a clean bowl, beat egg whites until soft peaks form.

2. Gradually add sugar and vanilla, beating until stiff peaks form.

3. Spread meringue over pudding.

4. Bake at 350°F for 12–15 minutes, or until lightly browned.

93 Cold Banana Pudding

Ingredients:

- 1 small box vanilla instant pudding
- 1 can sweetened condensed milk
- 1 box vanilla wafers
- 4 bananas, sliced
- 1 small container Cool Whip

Instructions:

1. Prepare pudding according to package directions.
2. Stir in sweetened condensed milk.
3. Fold in Cool Whip.
4. In a serving dish, layer cookies and bananas.
5. Spread pudding mixture on top.
6. Chill until ready to serve.

94 Four Layer Delight

Layer 1 (Crust) Ingredients:

- 1 cup flour
- 1 cup chopped pecans
- 3/4 cup brown sugar
- 1/2 cup butter

Instructions:

1. Preheat the oven to 350°F.
2. Mix crust ingredients and press into a pan.
3. Bake for 20 minutes and cool.

Layer 2 Ingredients:

- 1 large Cool Whip
- 1 large package cream cheese
- 1/2 box confectioners' sugar

Instructions:

1. Mix together and spread over the cooled crust.

Layer 3 Ingredients:

- 1 package instant Jello pudding (any flavor)

Instructions:

1. Prepare pudding and spread over cream cheese layer.

Layer 4 Ingredients:

- 1 small Cool Whip

Instructions:

1. Spread over the pudding layer.

2. until set and ready to serve.

95 Shoney's Strawberry Pie

Ingredients:

- 3/4 cup sugar
- Pinch of salt
- 3 tablespoons cornstarch
- 1/2 teaspoon red food coloring
- 1 cup + 2 tablespoons water
- 1 pint sliced strawberries
- 1 tablespoon lemon juice

Instructions:

1. In a saucepan, combine sugar, salt, and cornstarch.
2. Stir in water and bring to medium heat, stirring until thickened.
3. Add food coloring and lemon juice. Let cool.

4. Add sliced strawberries and stir gently.
5. Pour into a pre-baked pie shell.
6. Top with Cool Whip (optionally add a drop of vanilla to the Cool Whip for a homemade taste).

96 Louisiana Tater Pie

Ingredients:

- 2 medium sweet potatoes
- 1/2 stick margarine
- 1 cup sugar
- 1 1/2 to 2 teaspoons allspice
- 1 cup evaporated milk (Pet milk)
- 2 well-beaten eggs

Instructions:

1. Peel and slice sweet potatoes. Cook in a small amount of water, or boil whole and peel afterward.
2. Mash the cooked potatoes.
3. Stir in margarine and sugar while potatoes are still hot.
4. Once margarine melts, add allspice, milk, and

eggs.

5. Beat mixture well; it should be soupy.

6. Pour into an unbaked pie crust.

7. Bake at 400°F for 30 minutes.

97 Coconut Custard Pie (Diabetic-Friendly)

Ingredients:

- 2 2/3 cups skim milk
- 5 eggs
- 1 tablespoon Sucaryl solution or 24 Sucaryl* tablets, crushed
- 1/4 teaspoon salt
- 1 teaspoon vanilla. Dash of nutmeg
- 3/4 cup toasted coconut

Note: Sucaryl is a vintage artificial sweetener. For a modern substitute, consider using Stevia, Splenda, or your preferred sugar alternative.

Instructions:

1. Scald the milk in a saucepan (heat just until tiny bubbles form around the edge).
2. In a mixing bowl, combine eggs, Succaryl, salt,

and vanilla. Blend well.

3. Slowly pour the hot milk into the egg mixture while beating slightly.

4. Pour into a pre-baked Dieter's Pie Crust.

5. Sprinkle the top with nutmeg.

6. Bake at 450°F for 5 minutes, then reduce heat to 350°F and bake for another 15 minutes, or until a knife inserted near the center comes out clean.

7. Let cool, then garnish with toasted coconut.

98 Dieter's Pie Crust

Ingredients:

- 1/3 cup sifted all-purpose flour
- 2 tablespoons shortening
- 1/8 teaspoon salt
- 1/2 cup cottage cheese

Instructions:

1. Squeeze excess moisture from cottage cheese using a cloth, then press through a sieve.
2. In a bowl, cut shortening into flour and salt as you would for traditional pie crust.
3. Add cottage cheese and mix lightly with a fork until a dough ball forms.
4. Roll dough on a lightly floured surface to fit an 8- or 9-inch pie pan.
5. For a baked shell, bake at 400°F for 20 minutes.

99 Apple Pie

Ingredients:

- 5 cups sliced apples (about 5 medium apples)
- 2 teaspoons quick-cooking tapioca
- 1 tablespoon Sweet'N Low (or 14 packets)
- Ground cinnamon (optional)
- 2 recipes Dieter's Pie Crust (see above)

Instructions:

1. Roll out two-thirds of the pie crust to line an 8- or 9-inch pie pan.
2. Arrange sliced apples in the crust.
3. Sprinkle with tapioca, Sweet'N Low, and cinnamon if desired.
4. Roll out remaining crust, cut slits for steam, and place over apples.
5. Crimp edges and moisten with water if needed.

6. Bake at 400°F for 30 minutes, or until apples are tender.

100 Tapioca Pudding

Ingredients:

- 1 cup whole milk
- 1 tablespoon quick-cooking tapioca
- 1/4 teaspoon vanilla extract
- Sweet'N Low to taste
- Green food coloring (optional)

Instructions:

1. In the top of a double boiler, mix milk and tapioca.
2. Heat just until the milk begins to boil.
3. Remove from heat and stir in vanilla, Sweet'N Low, and a drop of food coloring if using.
4. Chill in the refrigerator before serving.

101 Strawberry Cheesecake

Ingredients:

- 1 1/2 cups cottage cheese
- 3 eggs
- 1/2 teaspoon almond extract
- 1 teaspoon Sweet'N Low (or 4 1/2 packets)
- Fresh strawberries, for garnish

Instructions:

1. Press cottage cheese through a sieve, then blend until smooth.
2. Beat in eggs, almond extract, and Sweet'N Low until creamy.
3. Pour into a buttered 9-inch layer pan.
4. Bake at 350°F for 20–25 minutes.
5. Cool completely, then top with fresh strawberries and a sprinkle of Sweet'N Low.

102 Whoopie Pies

Filling Ingredients:

- 1 cup confectioners' sugar
- 1 cup shortening
- 2–3 drops vinegar
- 5 teaspoons flour
- 1 cup milk (added slowly)

Instructions:

1. Mix all ingredients together.
2. Gradually add milk while beating until stiff.

Cookies Ingredients:

- 2 3/4 cups flour
- 1 teaspoon baking powder
- 1 teaspoon baking soda

- 1 tablespoon vanilla extract
- 1/2 cup shortening
- 1 1/2 cups sugar
- 2 eggs
- 1/2 cup sour milk
- 1/2 cup cocoa mixed with 1/2 cup hot water

Instructions:

1. Preheat the oven to 350°F.
2. Mix all ingredients until well blended.
3. Shape dough into golf ball-sized balls and place on a baking sheet.
4. Bake for 10 minutes. Do not over-bake.
5. Cool completely.
6. Spread filling on one cookie and top with another.
7. Wrap in plastic for storage or gifting.

103 Blueberry Pudding Cake

Fruit Layer Ingredients:

- 2 cups blueberries
- 1/2 teaspoon cinnamon

Batter Ingredients:

- 1/2 cup sugar
- 3 tablespoons butter
- 1/2 cup milk
- 1 cup flour
- 1 teaspoon baking powder
- 1/4 teaspoon salt

Topping Ingredients:

- 1/2 cup sugar
- Dash of salt

- 1 tablespoon cornstarch
- 1 cup boiling water

Instructions:

1. Preheat the oven to 375°F. Grease an 8x8 baking dish.
2. Spread blueberries in the bottom and sprinkle with cinnamon.
3. Cream butter and sugar. Stir in milk, then mix in dry ingredients.
4. Spread batter over the berries.
5. Combine sugar, salt, and cornstarch for topping. Sprinkle over batter.
6. Slowly pour boiling water over the top—do not stir.
7. Bake for 1 hour. Serve warm with Cool Whip or vanilla ice cream.

104 Old Time Rice Pudding

Ingredients:

- 1/2 cup rice
- 4 cups milk
- 1/3 cup sugar
- 1/2 teaspoon salt
- 1 teaspoon lemon juice
- 1/4 teaspoon nutmeg
- 1/2 cup raisins

Instructions:

1. Preheat the oven to 300°F.
2. Combine rice, milk, sugar, and salt in a greased 1 1/2-quart baking dish.
3. Bake for 1 hour, stirring several times.
4. Stir in lemon juice, nutmeg, and raisins.

5. Continue baking for 2 to 2 1/2 hours, or until thickened.

105 Cherry Coffee Cake

Cake Ingredients:

- 1 stick oleo* (or butter)
- 1 cup sugar
- 2 eggs
- 1 teaspoon vanilla extract
- 2 cups flour
- 2 teaspoons baking powder

Topping Ingredients:

- 1/3 cup flour
- 1/4 cup sugar
- 3 tablespoons oleo*
- 24 oz cherry pie filling

Instructions:

1. Preheat the oven to 350°F and grease an 8x11-inch pan.

2. Cream butter, sugar, eggs, and vanilla together.

3. Mix flour, and baking powder, then add alternately with milk.

4. Spread half the batter in the pan.

5. Pour cherry pie filling over the batter.

6. Add remaining batter on top.

7. Mix topping ingredients until crumbly and sprinkle over the cake.

8. Bake for 1 hour, or until golden and set.

106 Shortbread Cookies

Ingredients:

- 1 stick oleo*
- 1 stick butter
- 1/2 to 3/4 cup sugar
- 2 1/4 cups flour (added 1 cup at a time)

Instructions:

1. Preheat the oven to 350°F.
2. Cream together oleo and butter.
3. Add sugar and cream well.
4. Gradually add flour, mixing thoroughly.
5. Divide dough into 4 parts and pat each into a circle about 1/4 inch thick.
6. Cut each circle into 8 wedges.
7. Place on an ungreased baking sheet and bake

until light brown.

107 Tea Scones

These cookies were a favorite made by Ma Fitzgerald—low in sugar, but rich in love.

Ingredients:

- 2 cups self-rising flour
- 2 tablespoons sugar
- 1/3 cup currants (optional)
- 6 tablespoons oleo*
- 1 egg, beaten
- 1/2 cup milk

Instructions:

1. Preheat the oven to 425°F.
2. In a bowl, stir together flour and sugar. Add currants if using.
3. Cut in butter until the mixture resembles

coarse crumbs.

4. Add egg and milk, stirring just until dough forms.

5. Knead gently on a lightly floured surface 12 to 15 times.

6. Divide dough in half. Pat or roll each half into a 6-inch circle about 1/2 inch thick.

7. Cut each circle into 6–8 wedges.

8. Place on an non-greased baking sheet without sides touching.

9. Brush with beaten egg.

10. Bake for 12–15 minutes or until deep golden brown.

Index

1 Fried Chicken

2 Oven Fried Chicken

3 Skillet Pies

4 Chicken and Noodles

5 Chicken Spaghetti

6 Gumbo

7 Baked Chicken or Turkey

8 Aunt Modean's Stuffed Dumplings

9 Chicken Casserole

10 Giblet Gravy

11 Cornbread Dressing

12 Breasts Baked in Mushroom Sauce

13 Hot Chicken Salad Casserole

14 Chicken and Dumplings

15 Squirrel with Brown Dumplings

16 Hobo Beans

17 Teriyaki Chicken

18 Liver and Onions

19 Baked Chicken

20 Shrimp Creole

21 Shrimp Étouffée

22 Hamburger Steaks

23 Dirty Rice

24 Taco Casserole

25 Wilted Salad

26 Coleslaw

27 Overnight Salad

28 Chicken Salad

29 Potato Salad

30 Carrot-Raisin Salad

31 Green Pea Salad

32 Dry Beans

33 Bean Dumplings

34 Corn Pudding

35 Candied Sweet Potatoes

36 Fried Green Tomatoes

37 Green Peas & Potatoes

38 Broccoli Casserole

39 Green Bean Casserole

40 Sweet Potato Casserole

41 Mixed Squash Casserole

42 Tater Tot Casserole

43 Canned Green Beans

44 Turnip Greens and Corn Dodgers

45 BISCUITS

46 MEXICAN CORNBREAD

47 BANANA BREAD

48 LEMON GLAZED BREAD

49 BLUEBERRY MUFFINS

50 MONKEY BREAD

51 HOT WATER CORNBREAD

52 CAN BISCUIT CINNAMON ROLLS

53 CAN BISCUIT DONUTS

54 MAMA PETTY'S HUSH PUPPIES

55 IRISH SODA BREAD

56 PUMPKIN BREAD

57 SWEET APPLE QUICK BREAD

58 DATE NUT BREAD

59 Strawberry Angel Food Cake

60 Easy Cake

61 Grandma Petty's Stack Cake

62 German Chocolate Upside Down Cake

63 Fruit Cake

64 Ultimate Carrot Cake

65 Chewy Cake

66 Italian Cream Cake

67 Lemon-Jello Cake

68 Mandarin-Orange Cake

69 Mississippi-Mud Cake

70 Orange Slice Cake

71 Moist Pineapple Cake

72 Blueberry Pound Cake

73 Fresh Apple Cake

74 Better Than Everything Cake

75 Baked Apple Squares

76 Lemon Pound Cake

77 Honey Bun Cake

78 Baked Cheesecake

79 Orange Cake

80 Tunnel of Fudge Cake

81 Lazy Man's Peach Cobbler

82 Easy Apple Dumplings

83 Bread Pudding with Lemon Sauce

84 Butternut Brownie Pie

85 Pecan Pie

86 Pie Crust for Single Pie

87 Blind bake

88 Best-Ever Apple Pie

89 Hot Apple Toddy

90 Fried Apple Pies

91 Pastry (Double Pie Crust)

92 Banana Pudding (Custard-Based)

93 Cold Banana Pudding

94 Four Layer Delight

95 Shoney's Strawberry Pie

96 Louisiana Tater Pie

97 Coconut Custard Pie (Diabetic-Friendly)

98 Dieter's Pie Crust

99 Apple Pie

100 Tapioca Pudding

101 Strawberry Cheesecake

102 Whoopie Pies

103 Blueberry Pudding Cake

104 Old Time Rice Pudding

105 Cherry Coffee Cake

106 Shortbread Cookies

106 Shortbread Cookies

Acknowledgements

This book is a tribute to the love and legacy of **Sherry Fitzgerald Thorne**, and it would not be complete without honoring the many people who filled her life with meaning, laughter, and support.

To those who stood closest to her heart, thank you for being part of her story:

Gerald Lynn Thorne, Bubba Thorne, Candida Thorne, Aubrey & Thera Fitzgerald, Annie Mae & Bill Petty, Linda & Junior Snipes, Terry & Willie Fitzgerald, Pam Ammons, Michael Fitzgerald, Amy Sharp, Stacy Lee, Greg Gilley, Cole Thorne, Jessica Allan, Brooklyn Cutshaw, Hannah Thorne, Noah Thorne, and Zoe Tweed, each of you carried a piece of her love and light.

To **Momma's bunch of Yorkies**, who never left her side and brought joy to her every day, thank you for being her faithful little shadows.

And to **every person she met across the world**—from neighbors to friends, from distant relatives to strangers—who ever shared a recipe, a kitchen tip, or a better way to stir, season, or serve: your wisdom helped shape the pages of this book and the meals that came from her stove.

Sherry believed that good food was meant to be shared. So was kindness. This book is for all of you.

With love and gratitude,□
Todd Thorne

About the author

About the Writer

Sherry Fitzgerald Thorne was a mother, a sister, a grandmother, an aunt, and a true Southern soul whose love flowed from her kitchen into the hearts of everyone around her. She was the proud mother of two boys and a loving sister to both a brother and a sister. Her life was shaped not only by the family she raised, but by the extended family she cherished; nieces, nephews, and grandchildren who all felt her warmth, her wisdom, and her unwavering affection.

Sherry was born and raised in **Monroe, Louisiana**, where her roots took hold in the red clay and magnolia-scented air of the Deep South. Later, she made her home in **Greeneville, Tennessee**, where her heart settled into the rhythm of Appalachian hills and seasons. She spent many of her happiest years atop a large hill in **Rheatown, Tennessee**, in a weathered old farmhouse with a sprawling kitchen and an even larger dining room.

It was there, in that home on the hill, that Sherry became the center of so many family memories. On holidays like Thanksgiving and Christmas, the table was always full of food, of stories, of laughter. Her cooking brought everyone together, and her home was a place where people came not just to eat, but to feel seen, known, and loved.

She lived simply, loved deeply, and gave generously, especially when it came to feeding those around her. This book, like the meals she made, is a gift from the heart. A reflection of who she was. A legacy that continues to nourish.

Made in the USA
Monee, IL
11 November 2026

900c8ff3-1d5b-4760-b184-e8a24c4b2686R01